Intermittent Fasting Complete Beginners Guide to Intermittent Fasting to Rapidly Lose Weight, Heal Your Body, and Burn Fat ....

About Hirouchi Jeson

Hirouchi Jeson has a degree in biology from St. Thomas University in St. Paul, Minnesota. For more than 34 years, he has worked in the fields of medicine and healthcare to bring to the market new FDA-approved therapies and technologies that specialize in the heart and brain. Hirouchi is currently Vice President of Sales for the Neurovascular Division of a major US healthcare company.

As a busy leader in the field of medical devices and having a demanding career, Hirouchi has discovered the secrets of what it takes to live a vibrant and fulfilling life. Hirouchi has been married and happy for over 25 years. He raised three daughters with his wife and enjoys living in Southern California as a passionate surfer. Hirouchi is often described by those who know him best as an innovator, highly motivated, funny and someone who never takes "No" as an answer.

After being questioned about a million times about how he manages to stay in such good shape, author Hirouchi Jeson decided to share his passion for life thoroughly and reveal a secret he discovered.

Hirouchi says, "I did not have time to exercise or diet, I just had time not to eat, to fast at work." Hirouchi shares the story of his successful fasting weight loss, his three personalized and proven fasting methods, and the many health benefits of what was discovered as a natural way of eating.

For more information contact Hirouchi at :
hj@HirouchiJeson.com

INTRODUCTION

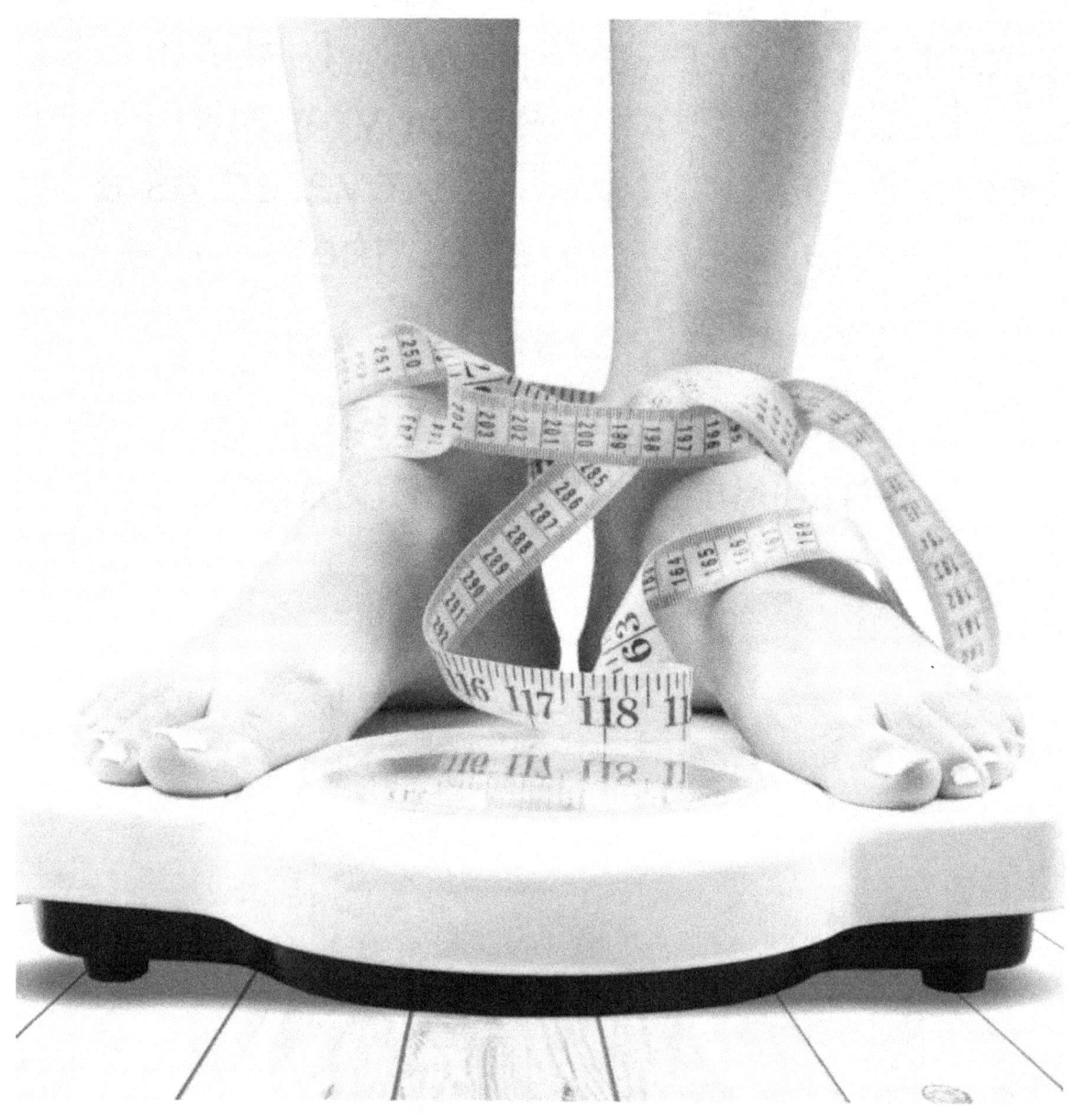

If you are interested in fasting for weight loss but don't have time to do it long-term, then this BOOK will strip you of that excuse and - hopefully - move you into action. Enough is enough. The time is NOW to lose excess weight and cleanse your body dear friend.

Life is too short. Let us not allow any more precious time to pass in obesity and sickness.

Why not try intermittent fasting? Some people think that unless they fast for days and days, then they might as well not do it at all. That is just not the case. In fact, fasting intermittently can be just as powerful. It can hold incredible health benefits for you; in mind, body and spirit. Any period of time that the digestive system can get to rest and focus on cleansing will help you.

If your boss tells you that "you can go home for the day." Will you refuse because he isn't giving you the entire week off? Or will you jump at the chance to rest even for a few hours? Of course! You would go home, right? Well, so is the digestive system. It will be VERY grateful for the rest, even if you stop eating only for a few hours. THAT is at the very heart of what intermittent fasting is all about.

Intermittent fasting means means that you will select certain hours and/or days during which you will not eat solid food. Instead, you can drink water or juice - depending on the type of fast you wish to do. Fasting with water only will provide greater weight loss but is also more difficult.

So if you are a beginner, I suggest you start with a juice fast. Better to put the fruit low so you can reach it. In other words, make it easy for yourself. You can always fast for longer periods of time later if you wish. Always remember: slow is fast. This is not a race.

That's why intermittent fasting is such a great way to go. Perhaps not everyone can fast for 30 days, but pretty much everyone can skip a meal several times a week, or fast for a 24-hour cycle. It doesn't matter whether you have successfully fasted in the past or not, this type of alternating structure can work for you. It wipes away any fears and/or excuses you might have had for not taking action.

Let's look at several intermittent fasting methods that you can consider.

The easiest way to start is by simply skipping a meal three times per week (or even every day)... usually lunch. When you wake up, eat your breakfast as usual. You can then fast through lunch and break the regimen at night with a sensible dinner. This is similar to the type of fast many do during the lenten season. They fast from sunup to sundown every day for 40 days. Why don't you give that a shot?

Another option is to fast for 24-hours (from 8am to 8am, for example) followed by 24 hours of normal (but improved health-wise) eating. You would, in essence, be fasting "every other day." Some people do this indefinitely until they reach their weight loss and/or health goals.

Let's go a bit further. You can also fast for half the week, meaning (for example) that you would have breakfast Monday morning and then fast through Thursday evening. How does that sound? You would break the fast with a light salad, steamed veggies and/or fruit.

Slightly harder but very powerful is weekly intermittent fasting. In other words, you fast from Sunday to Sunday, then you return to eating for the same number of days, and then resume fasting. So you would be fasting "every other week" for an entire seven days. One man I coached some time ago followed this system for six months and lost 145 pounds.

So what are you going to do? While a regular fast may not be for you, I am certain that doing it intermittently is something that you CAN do. Even skipping one meal every few days is better than doing nothing. The journey of a thousands miles begins with the first step, right?

Or perhaps you are afraid of fasting. Yes, I can understand. There are a LOT of misconceptions out there about this discipline. Some people may tell you that you will "die" if you do not eat every day. Or that your body will collapse for lack of nutrition. To be sure, I DO recommend that you first get a checkup if you are unsure about your health. However, in most cases, fasting does not deteriorate health. Rather, it improves it!

The bottom line is that you're not alone. There are many out there that are adopting this amazing discipline and seeing remarkable results. Think about what your motivations are. Why do you want to fast? What do you think you'll gain from it? Cementing your goals and motivation in your mind can help you follow through with it.

Don't let this be just another article you read on your path to losing weight and getting healthier. Make this "the day" you decide to start to walk towards your health and weight loss goals. There are literally no excuses for not making this a priority. What can be more important than your own health?

What will happen to your loved ones if you become ill? What price are you willing to pay in your mind and body for NOT taking action? I submit to you that whatever hunger or discomfort we go through while fasting is little in comparison to the HUGE health benefits we receive. You can see permanent change in your life. You can make this happen! Start today... how about right now?

This book is to provide a little bit of an over view about Intermittent Fasting and what it is all about. This isn't a how to, tell all or prescription on how to do an intermittent fast, more so just to answer some of the questions I have been receiving on this newest of the "weight loss systems" that is creating a buzz.

What is Intermittent Fasting

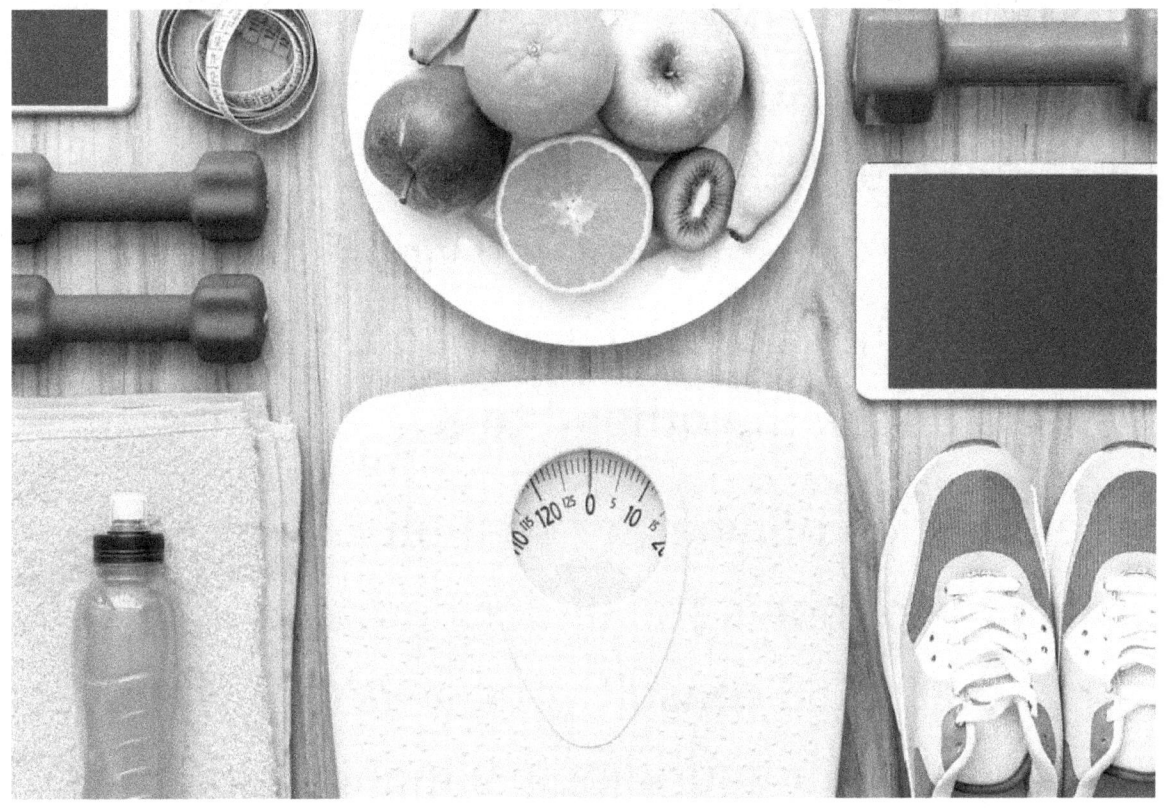

What is intermittent fasting?

It is an eating patter where one fasts for a set period of time and then eats for another set period of time. The three most common approaches that I have seen in the literature are the once a week/month, 24 hour and the daily 16/8 or 20/4 intermittent fast. During the 24 hour routine, the individual doesn't eat or drink anything with the exception of water, green tea and maybe some Branch Chain Amino Acids (BCAA) for a 24 hour period. Then, after that 24 hour period has expired they begin eating again. During the 16/8 or 20/4 routine, the individual does not eat for either 16 to 20 hours and then eats meals during the other 4 to 8 hour period.

The question of whether an intermittent fast is healthy or not is still undecided, and that is why you should consult your physician when wanting to alter your diet in a manner such as this.

Will I lose weight doing an intermittent fast? This is also a very debatable question, because it really depends on many other mitigating factors such as, what is your "normal" non fasting diet consisting of, do you have any underlying medical issues etc... If you fast for one day, but your diet consists of nothing but processed foods, fast food, animal products and desserts then no, your probably not going to lose weight. One must have a sound base of nutritional knowledge before they can use intermittent fasting as a weight loss system.

In general, this type of eating/fasting routine has been widely used by athletes, weight lifters and body builders as a way to "lean out" and decrease their body fat percentage. Those three groups all have one thing in common... they all understand the nuts and bolts of nutrition as well as the more advanced aspects of nutrition, so adding in something like the routines discussed above to lose a few percentage points off of their body fat and "lean out" is an easy addition to their routine.

Intermittent fasting weight loss is one of the most effective ways to shed off your extra pounds. The ideas on intermittent fasting weight loss challenge most of the previously held beliefs on losing. Those who are seeking new ways to lose weight effectively have Quickly embraced its ideas.

What is Intermittent Fasting Weight Loss?

Let me start by clarifying that intermittent fasting is not a diet. You are probably tired of trying anything with the word 'diet' on it when it comes to weight loss. Intermittent fasting is a way of eating that involves a structured program on the times when you eat and when you do not eat. You structure your program according to your fancy. If you can handle it, fast for a whole day! I recommend that you fast for 12 full hours before eating a meal. You can increase your fasting period later as you continue with the program.

What Makes it Different?

If you have tried to lose weight, you probably have tried diets such as Atkins diet based on the frequent feeding theory. Simply, proponents of such diets told you to eat often during the day. The idea was that the more you eat, the faster your metabolism. The faster your metabolism, the more fat you will lose. Of course, you do know that the more you ate, the more you wanted to eat and the more your weight remained. When you are on an intermittent program, you will have to cut down your meal frequency. Sometimes, you have to do without breakfast.

Tell Me More

You probably sleep for around 6 to 8 hours. During this time, your body is in fasting mode. When your body is in fasting mode, it usually produces more insulin. More insulin in your body causes your body to have increased insulin sensitivity. When your body has increased insulin sensitivity, you lose more fat. The brilliance of intermittent fasting weight loss program is that you skip breakfast to extend the period of your body's insulin sensitivity. This means that your body is going to be on fat loss mode for a longer period. You will lose more weight.

A longer fasting mode also has a good effect on the Growth hormone levels in your body. By skipping breakfast or eating during a specific period, your body produces Growth hormone. Growth hormone is what you want your body producing when you are trying to lose weight. This is simply because Growth hormone promotes weight loss in your body. When you are on an intermittent fasting weight loss program, your Growth hormone levels are usually at their peak. You will be losing more weight during this period. High

Growth hormone levels in your body also have several other health benefits. This program is simply amazing!

Intermittent fasting weight loss program is radically different from most weight loss programs being promoted in the market. However, its ideas are scientifically sound when it comes to losing weight. You should give this program a go if you are serious about weight loss.

Intermittent fasting has become quite the phenomenon these days. Recent studies showed that people who tried it have lost weight, increased health, and believed to have a long lifespan. Basically, intermittent fasting is a pattern of eating that alternates between periods of fasting, usually consuming only water, and non-fasting, usually eating anything a person want no matter how fattening. In other words, a person can eat anything he wants during a 24-hour period and fast for the next 24 hours. This approach to weight control seems to be supported by science, as well as religious and cultural practices around the globe. Adherents of intermittent fasting claim that this practice is a way to become more circumspect about food.

There are many different popular intermittent fasts and hundreds more possible variations. There are two kinds of intermittent fasts that are most basic and frequently used. First is the daily fasting in which the person only gets to eat once every 20-28 hours within a 4-hour period. The second is fasting for 1-3x a week, also called alternate day fasting, in which a person eats anything he wants on one day and fast the whole of next day.

Intermittent fasting has many beneficial effects as tested on animals like rodents and primates. One study found that there has been a "reduced serum glucose and insulin levels and increased resistance of neurons in the brain to excitotoxic stress". In 2008, a study on intermittent fasting showed that lifespan increases of 40.4% and 56.6% in C. elegans for alternate day (24 hour) and two-of-each-three day (48 hour) fasting, respectively, as compared to an ad libitum diet. And a 2009 study showed that intermittent fasting on rats improved long-term survival after chronic heart failure via pro-angiogenic, anti-apoptotic and anti-remodeling effects.

Researchers caution that only a few studies have been done on humans who are practicing intermittent fasts. The effects of exercise and meal frequency on body composition are an interesting but largely unexplored area of research. However, there are some positive results. Just last month, the Proceedings of the National Academy of Sciences published a study showing that reducing calories 30% a day increased the memory function of the elderly. In 2007, the journal Free Radical Biology & Medicine published a study that showed asthma patients who fasted had fewer symptoms, better airway function and a decrease in the markers of inflammation in the blood than those who didn't fast.

Complete Guide To Fasting Intermittent For Loss Weight

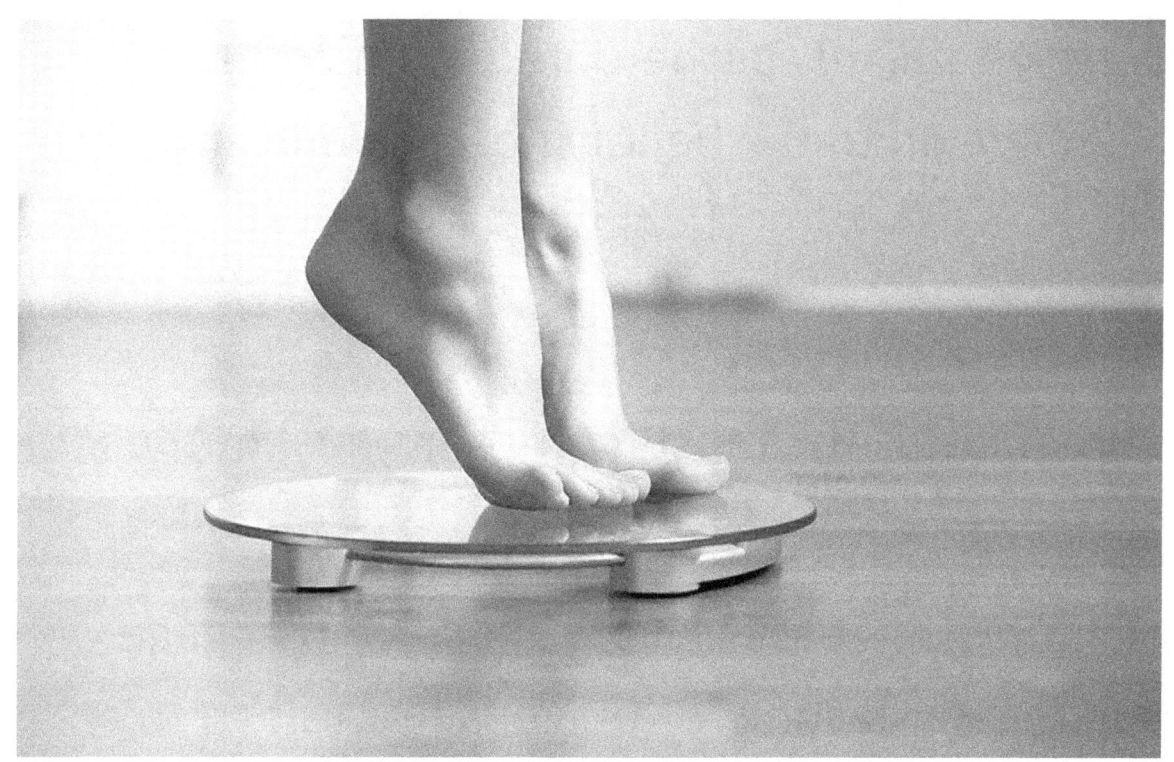

Everyone always wonders what the next big secret in the dieting industry is... Specifically, people want to burn fat and build muscle while putting in as little effort as possible. They want it all, and sometimes that's asking a little too much. At-least with most programs.

But what If I told you there were programs ahead of the entire industry that could do that? Enter intermittent fasting.

Let's kill a highly perpetuated myth before we move on to the benefits of intermittent fasting.

Breakfast is the most important meal of the day:

That myth is easily killed. Those who engage in regular fasting (often goes from sleep to lunch, meaning skipping breakfast) report increased focus, increased energy levels and better mood while fasting. Looking for your new coffee? You've found one that burns fat and gives you energy.

Eating 6 Meals A Day Speeds Up The Metabolism:

If you are consuming the same number of calories and have the same macronutrient distribution (primarily talking about protein), consuming those calories and nutrients between 6 meals and 1 makes near 0 difference. Because at the end of the day with either method, if I cut calories, there will be the same caloric deficit, and if I add calories, there will be the same surplus!

And if there was a difference, I am inclined to believe that it is in favor of the fasting method.

By increasing insulin sensitivity, intermittent fasting can make sure when you are eating the calories are getting driven directly into your muscles! And when you aren't fasting the increased adrenaline / noradrenaline will give you energy and burn fat!

In the most simple sense, intermittent fasting is rotating between periods of eating, and periods of not eating. I'll list the benefits below, but the general reasoning behind participating in Intermittent fasting(IF) is that many people respond very well to eating most of their calories in less meals, especially while dieting.

This allows for hunger control, insulin sensitivity (read: muscle building) and more time for burning fat (increased adrenaline/noradrenaline).

Methods:

You might fast through your sleep and into the afternoon, and then have a window of eating that lasts a few hours. In this period you would also have the workout.

Or it could mean that you wake up and eat a large meal, and fast late into the day until second/last meal.

Be smart and efficient, choose a program that gets you results with researched efficient methods. Either way the responsibility is taken at your leisure, but to squeeze the most results out of any method you choose, do your research and listen to your body.

Possible Benefits of Intermittent fasting:

Increased Insulin sensitivity/nutrient portioning, makes for a great way to build muscle without gaining fat!

Increased adrenaline/noradrenaline, meaning more time spent burning fat!

Reduced appetite and hunger, possibility of feeling full due to eating all calories in fewer meals

Example:

If you're allotted 1800 calories on your diet, would you rather eat 2 900 calorie meals, or 6 300 calorie meals?

Increased energy and focus

And so much more…

This is everything you want in a diet. We want to reap all the benefits while building the body of our dreams and this is the perfect way to do it! This is how you accomplish the number one goal of the fitness industry... burning fat while building muscle!

3 Main Reasons Why You Should Do It:

1. Maximum Fat Loss:

The main reason why you should do it is that intermittent fasting consumes maximum fats. Just imagine, if you implement fasting just for two days a week, you are cutting a whole full two days calorie quota from your weekly consumption! And this combined with your daily workout can give excellent results and you will loss excessive fat.

2. Maintains workout load very well:

The second reason for fasting is that it allows you to maintain a moderate to intense workout load without losing your energy and metabolism. Most of the people think that fasting drains your energy and metabolism but that's not true. If you implement fasting in your diet plan, you will get more energy and a higher metabolism.

3. Its Beneficial Aspects:

The third reason why the fasting is a good practice to include in your workout plan is its beneficial aspects which give you great benefits.

When you do any type of fasting, your body adjusts to it by consuming your body fat.

It also has some psychological benefits, like you would feel that you are not a slave to food.

A little disclosure:

Intermittent fasting is way ahead of the rest of the industry. It goes against a lot of the mainstream myths that are currently being perpetuated and that you might believe. But then again, we have to ask ourselves, do we want mainstream results? Or do we want to be above average, unique and at the top? I know my answer.

Therapy The Weight Problem

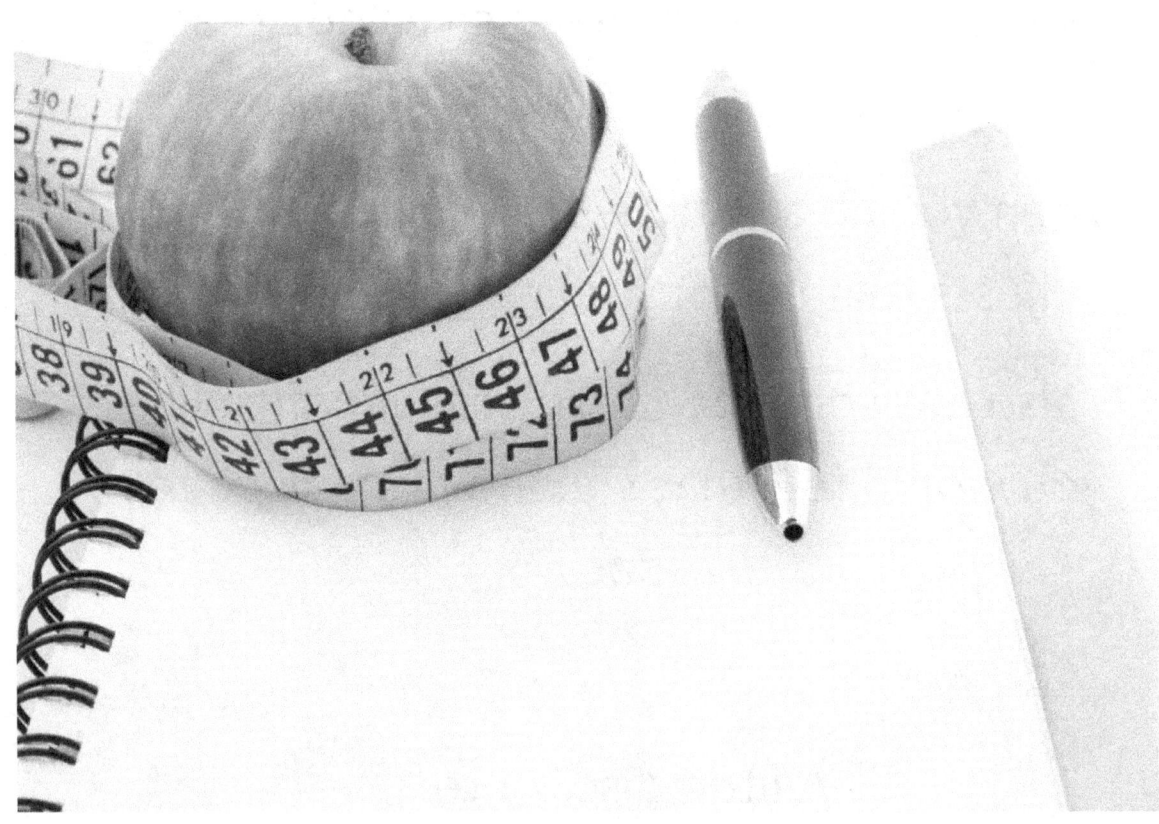

Health is wealth. It is described as the optimal well-being of an individual whether it is physical or psychological in nature. Staying fit and healthy promotes a positive outlook and maintains a youthful and vibrant disposition. Not only does it preserve youth, it also prolongs life. Now, one of the most innovative ways to keep oneself healthy and fit is through intermittent fasting. If you want to preserve your health, youth and the vitality of your being; then intermittent fasting should be given a try.

Intermittent fasting, as described today, is one of the cheapest fasting diets to lose weight. It doesn't require any other tools such as pills or medicines, nor does it entail any expensive gym equipment. All it simply asks is a strict and stern discipline to fasting. Intermittent fasting, by definition connotes the regulation of food intake by not ingesting anything between major meals. Also, by the word intermittent, it follows that a sequential order of eating pattern must be attained.

There's a presumption among experts that the basis on how intermittent fasting actually works can be explained by reason of anatomy and physiology; or the study of the organ and organ systems in relation to their functions within our bodies. As explained by specialists such as physicians, within our brain stem lies the seat of satiety, hunger and thirst called the hypothalamus. The hypothalamus is a complex, multifarious organ which actually orders our body when to feel the urge to gobble.

Hence, should there be any desire for man to drink or eat; the hypothalamus is the one responsible for such action. Thus, if left untrained and left to do on its own will, satiety and hunger will increase to huge proportions.

Once this happens, the urge to drink or eat will also be magnified. Of course, there is no danger or risk to eating. There is absolutely nothing wrong with that; however, the quality of the food intake we eat also determines the state of health among individuals. Likewise, if a person continually ingests foods that are not nutritious, say the one we see in fast foods or cafeterias; and done in large amounts, health is affected. Uncontrolled eating can lead to a host of diseases such as diabetes, hypertension, cardiac or heart problems and obesity.

The best way to start your fasting is to carefully plan your meals. Intermittent fasting works best if it is done regularly and habitually. This form of fasting diet to lose weight must be done in accordance with the willingness of the participant; and must be disciplined in order to achieve the desired effects. Aside from fasting, if you plan to lose weight, the amount of caloric intake must also be considered. So, aside from carefully planning the intermittent meals, the amount of calories must also be taken into consideration.

Combining the two strategies will not just make you slim; it will help you get the weight you've always wanted. Moreover, training your hypothalamus to eat intermittently will have a huge impact on your urge to eat or drink which would lead to restraining your unhealthy eating habits.

Today more and more people are paying attention to healthy eating diet guides. For some, it is about achieving their ideal body weight. For others, it is just about feeling and looking healthy both from inside and outside. As somebody put it rather well 'You are what you eat'. Think of what you made for supper - You knew that the casserole would be as good as the freshness and variety of ingredients you put into it. The human body is not different. It needs a selection of nutrients, vitamins and food groups to function well. If all it gets is processed and fried snacks and colas, you can well imagine the results.

Diet guides if followed for 5 days or 7 days a year like a detoxification program don't really help. You need to make changes that you can live with over a lifetime. So make them slowly, one vegetable at a time but at a pace where they become part of your life and not something that requires self-control. The goal should never be fast weight loss but a step towards your ideal body weight. Think of every morsel that you put as doing wonderful things for your body, chew it, savour the flavor and then swallow. How you eat is as important as what you eat, in order that it is assimilated. Some of the principles that I recommend as part of a diet guide as given below.

Eat Your Breakfast: Many people skip breakfast since they aren't really hungry or in a rush mistakenly believing that they have saved on calories. What they don't realize is that they have kept their basal metabolic rate low reduced alertness since the body has no fuel and multiplied their chances of overeating at lunch. By which time, the body will end up absorbing whatever it gets leading to higher chances of weight gain.

Focus On What You Are Eating: It is important to give food your complete attention while eating. Watching TV when eating or talking on the phone results in your brain not getting the 'I'm full' signals from your stomach making you consume more than what is required. Also it is believed that food is better metabolized if you focus on the eating process rather than elsewhere.

Eat Slowly: Chewing your food and eating it slowly helps you get the flavors giving you more satiety with lesser quantity. It also allows your brain to register fullness since the stomach takes some time to communicate this to the brain. If you're eating fast then you would have already overeaten by the time you get the message.

Eat More Frequently: Not many people realize that the very act of eating burns calories. Eating smaller meals serves two purposes. First it keeps the metabolic rate high so you burn more calories. Secondly by eating often, you prevent a situation where you 'react to food' or eat without thinking, often the reasons for eating extra.

Gap After Last Meal: Last but not the least remember to keep a gap of at least two hours between your dinner and sleep time. This will ensure that the meal gets metabolized well.

Reverse All diseases Chronic While Eat The Food You Like

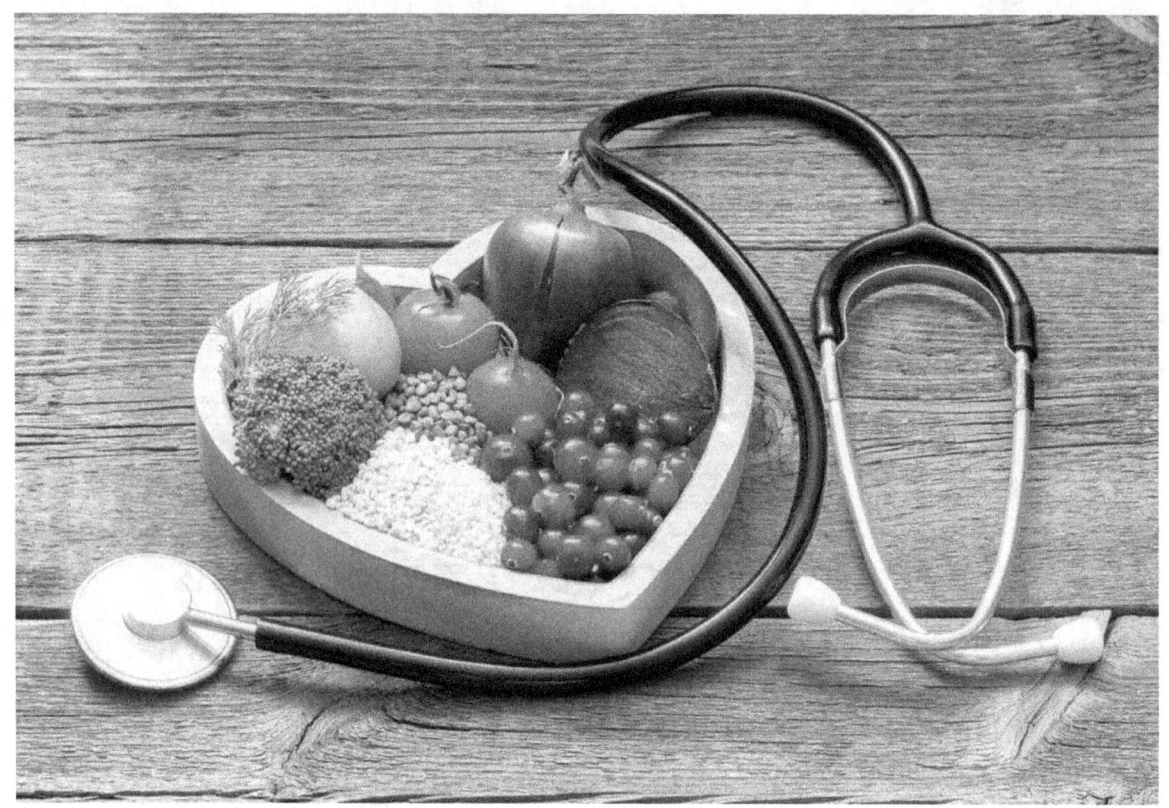

People argue that it is impossible to lose as much as 10 pounds in a week. One thing to bear in mind is that weight loss programs successes are relative. You can adopt a program that worked wonders for your friends but won't work for you. So it is always imperative to find and adopt a program that best suits you and that will keep you healthy too. You have to understand that the sole aim of every good weight loss program is not only to help you shed weight alone but also to help you stay healthy as well.

Home remedies for weight loss is a sure success for every one no matter how previous programs that do not work for you but worked for others. Natural remedies like reducing by at least 60% of your daily calories intake during your meals and burning 75% more is a very healthy approach. Reducing your calorie intake does not mean reducing the amount of food you eat. You can still eat the same amount of food. Starving yourself will only lead you to bigger health problems like ulcer and it will be in your best interest to stay off such approach as much as you can. You can continue eating and enjoying your meat but just cut the fat out and substitute meals like burger and steak with whole grain bread.

Consistency is the key to your diet program. Stick with the natural methods of reducing your weight. Taking a glass of water before meal, and taking fruits and vegetables in place of junk foods will really help you achieve your goals faster than you think. Cut down on the starch and sugars as much as possible. Alcohol should be eliminated just as caffeine should be eliminated. Undertake to walk at least 30 minutes because it helps to keep your body fit and healthy. Exercises such as jogging, biking, cycling should be done regularly and consistently. Ensure you have a particular time of the day that you these exercises (preferably in the morning) and you will be amaze at the kind of results you will get in a very short time of doing them. Losing 10 pounds in a week naturally is not impossible. Exercise regularly and balance it with a healthy nutrition and balanced diet and you will notice the amazing weight reduction.

10 TIPS FAST TO LOSE WEIGHT AND DIET

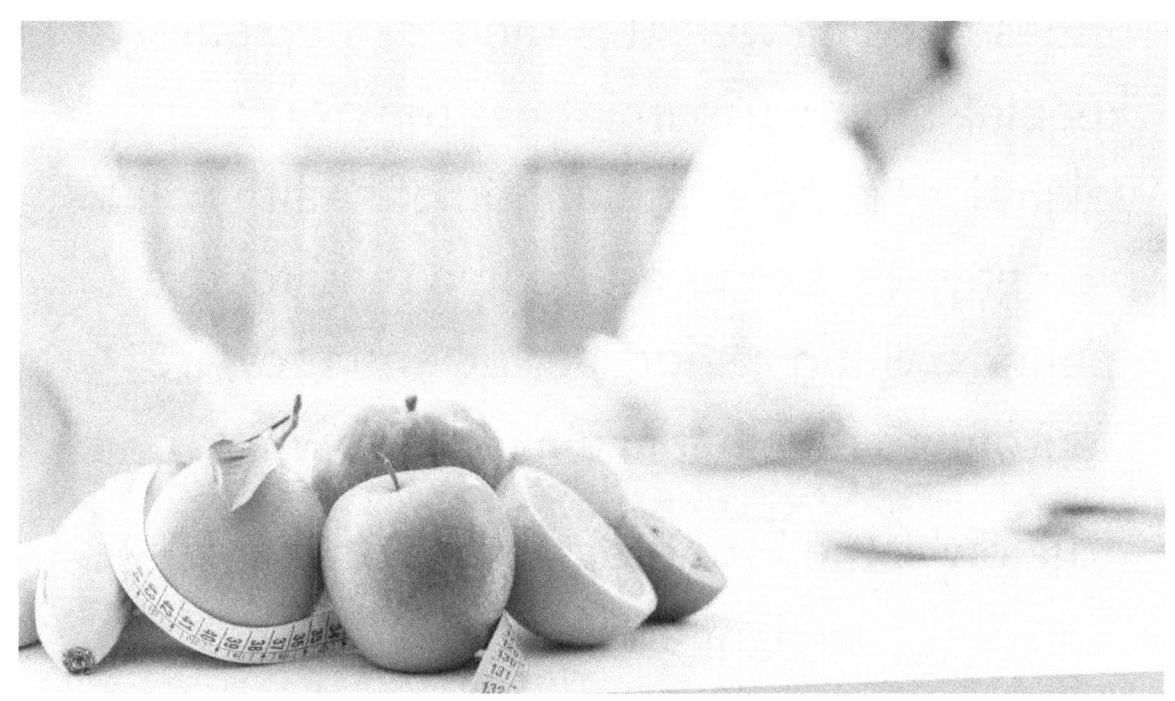

To lead a healthy long life, it is very certain to learn the facts about health, nutritious diet, and physical activities. The key for a healthy lifestyle is to know about eating right food and how to be physically active. An individual needs 30 minutes of physical activity at least 5 days a week. By avoiding illegal drugs and tobacco, the life span of an individual is sure to increase.

The most important thing in keeping healthy is losing the extra pounds and maintaining the weight. Out of every 3 Americans 2 are obese. Losing weight is the first step and keeping it off permanently is the next step. Weight loss is the combination of healthy diet and physical exercises. People tend to lose pounds within a short period and they are prone to regain it again in short while.

Below is the list of top 10 tips on losing weight and dieting.

Take regular exercise. Physical exercise has become the sole most effective fat burning enhancer around. The more you exercise the greater calories your body will burn up for energy. Performing some type of physical exercise, for example regular workouts to lose weight or simply a brisk walk several times weekly has been proven to be a very safe and natural way to speed up your metabolism Quickly.

Drink Green Leaf Tea. There is certainly some proof that consuming green tea will help you increase your metabolism. Certain chemical compounds such as a natural level of caffeine and catechin which is an anti-oxidant present in green leaf tea, have been proven to boost the level at which your body burns up calories. Green tea could possibly have significant benefits when it comes to weight reduction if it is consumed half an hour prior to an exercise routine.

Crash diet to lose weight is not the right way. By losing weight rapidly you are losing only the water content and glycogen and not fat. When you are in strict diet your body finds it difficult to burn calories. Once when you start eating normally your body starts to store as much as food into the fat cells that will result in regaining the lost weight.

Don't avoid breakfast in the name of dieting. Breakfast is the most important meal of the day that supports your body with necessary energy for the whole day. For those looking for weight loss it is an important advice not to skip breakfast.

Best plan for weight loss is to substitute food and not to eliminate food. Eat food with reduced fat and lower calorie. Replace junk food with fruits and vegetables that are low in calorie and rich in fiber.

Always eat natural food. Avoid processed food and food with additives. Eating natural food shows that you are in the right track for a long-term weight loss.

Avoid aerated drinks in your diet completely. By doing this an individual can save an average of 360 calories or even more every day. Fruit juices, whole milk and diet soda can add unwanted calories to your daily intake. Replacing whole milk with skim milk or soymilk can bring lot of difference. Make sure to drink at least 2 liters of water everyday. Water is essential for your body in fat burning process.

Don't overeat. Don't eat till your stomach feels full. Because nutrients in the food take time to enter bloodstream, and move to the nerve centers in the brain, which regulate appetite. Give your body a chance to feel that you had enough to eat by eating slowly.

Exercising is very important in weight loss plan. But it doesn't mean to spend 4 to 5 hours a day in gym. Select exercise options that can fit into life style.

Set realistic goals on weight reduction for a specific period of time.

CPSIA information can be obtained
at www.ICGtesting.com
Printed in the USA
LVHW061018190619
621688LV00017B/698/P